THE ELDER CLIFF 1.0

THE ELDER CLIFF 1.0

DON'T Lose Your Life To Caregiving

STELLA NSONG

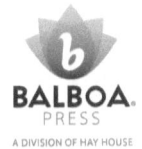

Copyright © 2013 Stella Nsong.

All rights reserved. No part of this book may be used or reproduced by any means, graphic, electronic, or mechanical, including photocopying, recording, taping or by any information storage retrieval system without the written permission of the publisher except in the case of brief quotations embodied in critical articles and reviews.

Author Credits: RN, CMC, CDP, LTCP

Balboa Press books may be ordered through booksellers or by contacting:

Balboa Press
A Division of Hay House
1663 Liberty Drive
Bloomington, IN 47403
www.balboapress.com
1-(877) 407-4847

Because of the dynamic nature of the Internet, any web addresses or links contained in this book may have changed since publication and may no longer be valid. The views expressed in this work are solely those of the author and do not necessarily reflect the views of the publisher, and the publisher hereby disclaims any responsibility for them.

Limits of Liability and Disclaimer of Warranty: The author and publisher shall not be liable for your misuse of this material. This book is strictly for informational and educational purposes.

Warning – Disclaimer: The purpose of this book is to educate and entertain. The author and/or publisher do not guarantee that anyone following these techniques, suggestions, tips, ideas, or strategies will become successful. The author and/or publisher shall have neither liability nor responsibility to anyone with respect to any loss or damage caused, or alleged to be caused, directly or indirectly by the information contained in this book.

Any people depicted in stock imagery provided by Thinkstock are models, and such images are being used for illustrative purposes only. Certain stock imagery © Thinkstock.

Printed in the United States of America.

ISBN: 978-1-4525-8199-6 (sc)
ISBN: 978-1-4525-8200-9 (e)

Balboa Press rev. date: 10/29/2013

CONTENTS

Introduction ix
About this Book xiii

Chapter 1: Why the Elder Care Cliff 1

    Top 10 Signs America is
    Facing an Eldercare Cliff . . . .
    See If You Agree! 4

**Chapter 2: What Other Caregivers Are
Saying! Do You Agree With
These Statements?** 7

Chapter 3: The AED Phases of Caregiving 19

    Top Seven Warning Signs
    and Symptoms of Caregiver
    Stress AKA Caregiver Syndrome 25

Chapter 4: Dying Early 29

    A True Story: Caregiver Dies
    Shortly After Her Dear Mother 31

    How Caregiver Stress Can
    Destroy You 36

Chapter 5: Measuring Your Caregiver Stress...... 41

    The Caregiver Syndrometer 43

    What Is the Level of Your
Caregiver Stress? 46

    The Caregiver Syndrometer
Scoring Checklist 47

Chapter 6: What Is Respite Care? 49

    The Three Most Common
Types of Respite Care Services 51

    How to Find "Quality" Respite Care 54

    Questions to Ask and What
to Look for When Hiring a
Private In-Home Caregiver 55

**Chapter 7: Ten Places to Get Money
and Resources for Respite Care** 57

**Chapter 8: The Five Components of a
Good Respite Plan** 67

    Where Can I Learn More
About Respite Services? 72

Chapter 9: Caring for Yourself So You Don't Die Early 75

  The Top 10 Ways to Care for Yourself .. 79

  The Thriving Caregiver's Declaration 83

Chapter 10: The Role of Care Management in Caregiving 85

  The Top 10 Ways a Care Manager Can Help with Respite Care .. 87

  The Three Best Places to Find Qualified Care Managers 88

Chapter 11: "Done for You" Respite Care Plan 91

  Respite Plan When You Have Less Than $100 per Month in Your Respite Budget 95

  Respite Plan When You Have $350 or More a Month in Your Respite Budget 97

  Tips about Respite Options 98

Chapter 12: The Six Steps to Making Decisions in Caregiving: The W.E.C.A.R.E. Model 99

    The W.E.C.A.R.E. Model: The Wheel to Drive Your Caring Situation 101

    Three Tips for Making Successful Decisions in Caregiving 104

    Beware of the "Shoulds" 105

About the Author 109

INTRODUCTION

My name is Stella Nsong and I am a caregiver. By education I am a registered nurse; earlier, I was a licensed practical nurse. I am also what people in the field of gerontology (the study of aging) call a certified geriatric care manager. Put simply, this means that I have a great deal of training, education and experience in caring for older adults, whom I like to address as the "mature and wise."

A few years ago I became a certified dementia practitioner, another fancy way of saying that I have been specially trained to care for someone with dementia—but more on that later.

In my personal life, I am a caregiver who is probably like you in some ways. Let me just stop here to say that I completely disagree with Merriam-Webster's definition of a *caregiver*. I am writing them a letter about that, and as soon as I get an answer, I will post it on my blog for you to see what they say about my strong opposition of their definition of **caregiver.**

According to Merriam-Webster.com, a caregiver is defined as:

> "a person who provides direct care (as for children, elderly people or the chronically ill)"

The dictionary also says that the first known use of the word *caregiver* was in 1966. So what did they call all those people who cared for the infirmed when my great grandparents where getting older? I know that they did not all do as the Eskimos did. Apparently, when you got older and became too much trouble, Eskimos took you and dropped you off somewhere on top of a mountain, and hoped to see you on the other side, if you can believe that.

You and I are real caregivers. Indeed, for the purpose of this book, caregivers are the people like you and me who do all of the following, plus a lot more:

- Make all the phone calls just to check in. It's either doing that or we worry ourselves sick about the safety and wellbeing of a loved one—and then we get busy looking for resources.
- We pick up the prescriptions, the newspaper, the garbage, the mail and sometimes the bills that we know nothing about.
- We do the hands-on care.

- We play nurse, transporter, cheerleader and wellness coach.
- We make the meals, do the laundry and cut the grass.
- We pay bills, file taxes and run the business.

For those of us who have managed to keep a job as well, we take time off work for the doctor appointments and the therapy sessions.

We get second-guessed, cursed out, slapped, kicked, accused and sometimes hugged, all of which can happen in the same day, and sometimes we get thanked for our help. We pay someone to be there to do these things when we are not able to be there.

We run all day, we worry in the process, we crash after midnight and we get up and keep doing the same, day in and day out. Sometimes we give all we have, 24 hours a day with days running into weeks and months and sometimes years. If you can relate to any of these scenarios, then this book is for you.

ABOUT THIS BOOK

The *Elder Care Cliff 1.0* is the first of a three part series of the *Elder Care Cliff* books. This book is about how not to die before the person that you are caring for dies. It is about taking time off for respite and self-care. It is about how respite care can save your life.

My goal here is to help you identify the areas of your caregiving situation that are the most stressful and damaging to your health, show you the importance of respite care, and guide you to formulate a respite plan for yourself and the person for whom you are caring, **so that you do not break down and die early**—perhaps even before the person you are caring for dies.

I have included a story that might make you cry, because it may hit too close for comfort in your situation. I tell this story to raise awareness that without taking time off and caring for themselves, caregivers can in fact die before their care recipients. I want to be your partner in caring for yourself when it is your turn to be a caregiver.

This book opens with an alarming summary of what I call the Elder Care Cliff. America is on the brink of a Caregiving crisis which deserves national attention. Approximately 65 million unpaid, overworked, and unrecognized family members in the United States find themselves thrust into the role of the family caregiver. By the year 2050, the elderly and infirmed in need of this care will outnumber those who will be able to provide the care. There is not one among us who will not be touched in some way by this health care dilemma. In the meantime, these invisible family heroes provide our entire healthcare system with a staggering amount of work and sacrifice that is beyond price. They need our help. Together we must face this challenge socially, politically, ethically and financially.

Chapter 2 introduces the importance of respite care for you, the family caregiver. The chapter begins with a letter from a client of mine who was contemplating suicide before he started taking time off for respite. The letter is followed by several quotes and comments, most of which came from family members of those that I have served and cared for in the last twenty years. Some came from members of my own family. The purpose of these quotes is to help you recognize that **you are part of a bigger circle of people with heart and people with patience:** that you are an artist performing the GREATEST ART OF LOVE . . . Caregiving.

Chapters 3-4 discuss the phases of caregiving, and the signs and symptoms of caregiver stress/caregiver syndrome. Chapter 5 offers you a guide to help you measure your caregiver stress. I have developed what I call the **caregiver syndrometer**—a gauge to measure your caregiver stress level. It is color coded, showing what is safe and what is dangerous, as far as the amount of stress that you are facing and dealing with. You will be able to measure your stress level in minutes. If your score is within the danger zone, I urge you to begin respite care right away so that you can start to lower your stress and your blood pressure, and guard your immune system.

Chapters 6-8 discuss the most common types of respite care services, the ten places to discover money and resources for respite care, and the components and essential elements of a good respite plan.

Chapters 9-12 are primarily about you. These are perhaps the most important parts of the entire book. They are about taking care of the most essential person in the care circle—you.

In Chapter 9, I have included the top ten ways to care for yourself, plus a declaration to your commitment to survive and thrive in caregiving. You should strive to do at least one of those ten actions each day. This may seem hard but once you make the commitment to care for yourself, you will see that your care recipient will also be taken care of. The life of the caregiver and the life of the care recipient are intertwined. When one is doing well, the other does well too and vice versa.

Chapter 10 introduces you to care management and the vital ways in which a care manager can assist you in your role as a family caregiver. You will learn exactly where to go to find qualified care managers.

In Chapter 11 you will find ready-made respite care plans to fit your budget and your needs.

Finally, you may feel like you and you alone carry the burden of making decisions for and about your loved one. This should never be the case. In Chapter 12, I give you a practical tool that will help you make *informed, shared* decisions in caregiving. I call it the W.E.C.A.R.E. Model. When followed, this model will become your source of confidence that you are giving the best care possible in the situation that you find yourself.

At the beginning of each chapter, I offer tips which I call *24/7 Lifeline Tips*. I hope these tips will serve as reminders for self-care, but I'm simply offering the tips as a way of supporting you so that you can survive and thrive in your role as a caregiver.

CHAPTER 1

WHY THE ELDER CARE CLIFF

* * *

24/7 Lifeline Tip #1

Regardless of generation we are all facing the elder care cliff. The secret to successfully bridge the cliff is to plan as a family unit, a work place issue and a national strategy.

* * *

The Elder Cliff 1.0

There are approximately 65 million unpaid family caregivers in America. If you are not an unpaid family caregiver, you most likely know one of them; they live in your city, on your street or even next door.

They serve with love, courage, never-ending patience and perseverance. They have mastered the art of juggling and balancing their multiple roles and responsibilities. Some work 24 hours a day with days blending into weeks, months and even years. Many of them have given up employment to attend to their loved ones, causing their own personal financial cliff. Adding insult to injury, most of the unpaid caregivers also have regular jobs and their taxes go to help fund some of the already limited care services for the aged, blind and disabled.

Today, these unpaid caregivers provide over $450 billion worth of care to their elderly parents and loved ones. This enormous sum is the cost of care and services that we working and tax paying people in America would otherwise have to pay, if these dedicated, courageous, resilient, unpaid family members were not available or willing to provide the care. Guess what would have happened to Medicare and Medicaid by now, if it were not for these family members whom I am going to call the invisible heroes of the U.S. healthcare system.

On behalf of all of us who recognize your importance and appreciate your dedication and your sacrifice, I Stella

Nsong would like to use this book to raise awareness of the fact that without these invisible heroes and without a solid plan for the eldercare system, America is facing a Caregiving crisis which I have decided to call the Elder Care Cliff. This is how the Elder Care Cliff series came about.

The Elder Care Cliff 1.0 is for the family caregiver. In this book, I discuss how to survive and thrive in Caregiving so that you do not lose your life to Caregiving.

The Elder Care Cliff 2.0 will be for the organizations who have Caregiving employees. That book will discuss what organizations can do to support their Caregiving employees, reduce their cost of work force retention and contain their health insurance utilization cost as it relates to family Caregiving.

The Elder Care Cliff 3.0 will discuss innovative ideas and collaborative initiatives between family caregivers, employers and policy makers so that together America can survive Caregiving to the year 2030 and beyond.

Top 10 Signs America is Facing an Eldercare Cliff . . . . See If You Agree!

- By the year 2030, the youngest baby boomers will turn 85.

- According to the Alzheimer's Foundation, 1 of 2 people aged 85 and older will suffer from Alzheimer's disease. Alzheimer's disease is the most expensive disease facing America today.
- A study conducted by the National Alliance for Caregiving in 2009 showed that there will not be enough people to care for seniors who are over 85 years of age—the fastest growing segment of the population. The population of people over 65 years of age is expected to increase at a rate of 2.3% but the number of family members available to care for them will only increase at a rate of 0.8%.
- In 2011, the Bureau of Labor Statistics conducted a study which revealed that one third of the population who are caregivers provide care for two or more people; 23% of the same population also cared for a minor child; 85% of these caregivers and their elderly loved ones did not live together; 56% of the caregivers were women and 44% were men.
- Today, there are about 5 people to provide care for an older adult but by the year 2030, research is showing that there will be only 3.6 persons and by 2050, there will be only about 2.9 persons available to care for an older adult.
- According to the *Evercare Survey of the Economic Downturn and its Impact on Family Caregiving*

in March 2009, family caregivers sustain the U.S. health care system with $450 billion of free care that they provide each year.
- According to *Assessment of Family Caregivers: A Research Perspective,* by Zarit, S. in 2006, 40% to 70% of family caregivers have clinically significant symptoms of depression, with approximately a quarter to half of these caregivers meeting the diagnostic criteria for major depression, yet go untreated. See the skyrocketing cost of the employer's health plan.
- According to the *MetLife Caregiving Cost Study,* it costs an employer an average of $2,300 per year per employee for loss of productivity associated with Caregiving. That is approximately $34 billion of potential loss to American businesses.
- America depends on the taxes of these employed caregivers so it can continue to fund the public and community services which are already limited and will be drastically reduced as the healthcare reform takes effect.
- It is the experience of the CAREgiving Institute in Painesville, Ohio that today, the family caregiver dies either before or shortly after the care recipient from stress related disorders associated with Caregiving or due to lack of self-care.

CHAPTER 2

WHAT OTHER CAREGIVERS ARE SAYING! DO YOU AGREE WITH THESE STATEMENTS?

* * *

24/7 Lifeline Tip #2

Alzheimer's disease is the third most expensive disease in the United States. More than 72% of people with Alzheimer's disease live at home and approximately 75% of their care is provided in the home by family members and friends. With the life expectancy increasing and the changes in the United States health care system, more care will be provided in the home—so get a respite plan in place. A respite plan is like a health care insurance plan. It takes care of you, and it helps you stay healthy so that you can continue to care when it is your turn to provide care.

* * *

THE ELDER CLIFF 1.0

In this chapter, I am calling all tired, exhausted, sometimes underappreciated and sometimes undercompensated caregivers—AKA the true INVISIBLE HEROS in the family—to see what others are saying about their situation.

I have picked nine quotes that deal with the most common aspects of caregiving, which are:

- Resistance to Care
- Anger
- Adapting
- Coping
- Decision Making
- Love and Loneliness
- Verbal Abuse
- Small Blessings, and lastly
- When Caregiving Becomes a Legal Issue

These quotes may help you realize what others are going through and to see how they deal with it. See if you can relate to any of these.

Resistance to Care

Below is a letter forwarded to me from a client named Marcus (I have his permission to use his real name). Marcus is not only terminally ill himself, but was contemplating suicide whenever he was not too busy providing care. That is how he spent his time before he started to get some respite care for himself and his loved one.

Marcus and his friend Mary, who lives in Georgia, share letters and stories about caregiving via email. Almost on a daily basis, these two caregivers share their lives through what has become an online support group for each other.

The letter below is from Mary to Marcus, and it was forwarded to me to keep me in the loop.

* * *

Friday morning, April 10th, 2010

Dear Stella,

My dearest friend Mary will often sign off as "Exit 72," an old and running joke linked to that exit on Interstate 44, for the town of Commerce, Georgia. Mary has been the End of Life scenario caregiver for three MD/PhD scientists at UGA, and is now on her fourth. Dr. Elareson, his wife Suzanne, his wife's sister (I forget her name) and her husband Jeff, who is currently in his last days, are the last of her caregiving commitments, or so she says.

The Elder Cliff 1.0

Her comments below will interest you:

Dear Marcus,

You've well-written another lively "review" of Stephen's caregivers. I'm sure Stella loves them.

I'm saddened to learn that Stephen HATES to get up, get clean etc. Does that mean he is so far gone and so depressed that he WANTS to stay in his bed all day and wait for death to join him? Does he later show any enjoyment of his time at the adult activity center? Does he ever laugh?

His threat of violent resistance reminds me of how Suzanne actually employed violence and physical non-cooperation suddenly after she became incontinent (urine only, thank god.) Her violence was limited to diaper-changing times. We had to INSIST that she allow us (me or Ann, the occasional "caregiver") to change her leaking, stinking diaper and wet slacks—a change which she could not accomplish alone. The procedure consisted of her lying on her back in bed, cooperating to lift her rump for me (or Ann) to pull off the wet stuff, and cooperating again to lift her butt to accept the dry diaper and fresh slacks.

Sometimes she would just refuse to lift her butt, but occasionally she would strike out with her fist or with her knee or with her feet. Poor John sometimes had to hobble in on his walker and bellow, "Suzanne, if you do not change your wet underwear, I will have to call the Health Department, and they may insist on taking you away." We did not know whether she understood the alleged choice, or whether it was just the scary BELLOWING, that made her submit in those instances to a change. Ann ($28/hour from a bonded agency) one day came out of Suzanne's room and said, "YOU go in there and change her. She SCARES me."

Whether Suzanne's Alzheimer's triggered both the incontinence and the anger, or if first the incontinence caused the rage at her fate, we'll never know. They were linked in time.

Is Stephen incontinent yet? Sooner or later, it is almost inevitable with dementia, I believe (Stella will have an opinion on that). Did any of Stephen's relatives show up, or was that a false alarm again? Helene never called me, so

I'm hoping that means her desperation has subsided a bit.

I'm doing my personal taxes, then the laundry and then preparing the snacks for tomorrow.

So, GOOD NIGHT! Much love, Exit 72.

Anger

"Sure, I get angry at Mary but that is part of being human. Sometimes she understands and sometimes she cries when she can see my anger. I just give myself time to cool off and then I remember what a wonderful woman she is and that helps me get over it. I just think that if she had her way, she would be taking care of me and that puts things in perspective for me."—Erni S.

Adapting

"There is nothing simple about caregiving. Several years ago, I would look at my neighbor and wonder what the heck has gotten into her. She would let her mother go outside in her house robe. Hell, I cried for the last two years over everything, I gained 60 pounds and ate 40 gallons of ice cream and ate myself into diabetes. Then I had a scare. I am now diabetic and stress was killing me.

"Suddenly, I began to see that life does not have to be that serious because the truth is, life goes on regardless of what was going on with me. I began to realize that using a towel more than twice was okay because after my shower, I was drying off water not dirt. That the grocery store opened 24 hours a day because it is okay to shop any day, anytime and the groceries will still be there if I don't go every Friday at exactly 11 AM. This new shift in attitude helped me lower my stress and I began to see things differently. All of a sudden, everything was not a big deal anymore and life went on and it is still going."—Miana M.

Coping

"I have reduced everything to two words: risk and benefits. What are the risks and how would it benefit me? Anything that does not fit in one of those categories gets thrown out and I am learning not to worry about what gets thrown out."—Deborah G.

Decision Making

"The best decision I ever made was to allow myself to get help when I was at the edge of a breakdown. One day in the middle of the afternoon I could feel myself almost suffocating in my own stress. My heart was beating so fast, I felt like the world was about to stop.

Asking for help was like the breath that I needed to save my life."—Bella N.

Love and Loneliness

"He did not speak for the 10 years following his stroke but he was at least here. Now that he is gone, I feel really lonely. I would rather him be here speechless and unable to walk. Though he wouldn't talk there was a sense of comfort of having him around."—Anne M.

Verbal Abuse

"My mom and I were never close. I left home as a teenager and now that she has dementia, it is hard to bond with her. She curses me especially in public. She talks about sex and having men coming into her house. Sometimes I feel that she knows what she is doing but I have passed the point of being mortified. I have learnt to laugh at her verbal abuse. Her doctor says that some of the cursing may be a result of a stroke and some of it was from dementia."—Marie J.

Small Blessings

"I have learnt that tomorrow is not a promise and that tomorrow things may be worse so today, I cherish what we have. If she can only remember my name or smile because she recognizes me then that is a blessing in itself. That thought helps me remain present in the moment. Now, I look out for moments because that is all that she is capable of. I collect moments and that helps me go from day to day."—Sheila N.

When Caregiving Becomes a Legal Issue

"I just slept nearly 12 hours. I am in very little physical pain now as I am currently taking prescribed Tramadol TID and 30mg of Oxycontin, BID. And the Neurontin seems to help some, but yesterday, nothing could have helped much. Got into bed, gave Miss Nibbles some KMFANR (you will recall, Kessler's Magic Fingers and Awesome Neck Rub), and promptly fell into a coma at 6:00 p.m.

"Sorry to hear about your diarrhea. Consider having David set up the telephone and computer in the bathroom, I mean, shit happens, but the least you can do between grunts is to use the time efficiently! Forgive me. I am trying to revive my ebbing sense of humor.

"This a.m., I awoke and began thinking about all this (as if I could think about anything else) and I am coming to the realization that my continuing to spend what time I have left trying to make sense out of insanity is simply not going to be my epitaph. I want out. And I am, as of today, going to begin taking steps to get the hell out. Tommy has agreed to reserve the next available apartment. I'll let you know.

"One sideline note here. Mother recently had a new will drawn up by another attorney, on her birthday, December 11th. The will specifies her four grandchildren as her heirs. You may recall that, in her original will, she made my brother and sister as the heirs leaving me out of it. This time she went a step further and had the attorney add a rather interesting clause. 'I am widowed. I have one living child, Marcus, and he has been purposefully and intentionally omitted from any gift or bequest under this my Will.'

"It is with nearly inevitable certainty that my mother will outlive me as her health and condition is less imminent or life threatening in the near term than mine. I have never been under any illusions about benefiting from my father's property because of that fact. Nevertheless, I have learned that there is a limit to my empathy and ability to disregard this kind of thing every time, trying to blame it on her disease. Right or wrong, Steinbeckian or not, this is simply not someone I want to help any further.

"My regret right now is that, by telling you all of this, you will feel compelled to respond. I cannot imagine how I would respond to such a thing, and to put you in that position, after all you have done for me, seems grossly unfair. There is nothing you can say. Your awareness is all I want because your letters have been a critically important outlet for my emotions and my creativity, and a little humor now and again. There simply isn't any price tag on that, so I would ask you NOT to try to respond to just this one unfortunate chapter. Next, I am working on a new commitment to me in my last days. It is funny to think that I am dying but I am also the caregiver to two people who do not care about me.

Love you,
Marcus"

* * *

My hope for you at this point of the book is that you will begin to formulate your own commitment to care for yourself. When you take care of yourself, you will realize that you will become a better caregiver in the process.

How do you take care of yourself? By making room in your life for **at least seven hours a day of respite time for you.**

CHAPTER 3

THE AED PHASES OF CAREGIVING

* * *

24/7 Lifeline Tip #3

The life of the caregiver and the life of the care recipient are intertwined. Taking time off for respite and having someone else provide care is an investment in your loved ones care. It is an act of love, not a denial of duty—so proudly give yourself permission to take time off for respite.

* * *

This chapter describes the typical patterns of how most family caregivers provide care, and what the family caregiver goes through before recognizing the need for outside help. It describes what I have determined to be the best names for each phase.

The phases of caregiving translate to the acronym of AED. No, not the AED (Automatic External Defibrillator) machine like you see at the airport that is used to shock a person when their heart stops. Although sometimes, I want to install a few of these machines in the homes of some of the families that I have worked with for fear that they might come in handy someday if the caregivers don't hurry and get some respite care.

The AED Phases of caregiving are:

- **A**daptation
- **E**xhaustion
- **D**amage and Irrecoverable

Adaptation Phase:

This is the first phase of caregiving. The time span is from one to 18 months.

In the adaptation phase, the caregiver is confident, feels as if he or she has everything under control, and family and friends are lending help when possible. This period of caregiving is also characterized by the care recipient being able to provide some amount of self care. Most of the time, there are no behavior challenges except for those instances where the care recipient is partially disclosing or not disclosing vital information or details critical to their independence and safety.

From the outside, most things appear normal except that the caregiver worries every now and then.

Exhaustion Phase:

This is the second phase of caregiving. The time span is usually between 19 months and 36 months. At this stage, the caregiver is now experiencing prolonged stress within his or her personal and work life. This period is characterized by the caregiver often taking medication for sleep or mood disorders.

During the exhaustion phase, the care recipient needs hands-on care and/or is suffering from some degree of self-care deficit. The caregiver's ability to cope is reducing and their social connections are weakening, so their support systems begin to fail. Outside help begins to diminish, except for errands, appointments and trips to the drug store or a grocery. This usually happens because friends and family members begin to see the quality of their relationship with the caregiver decline.

The caregiver begins to feel alone, isolated, depressed and physically ill. The caregiver's quality of work begins to diminish. Most are only working part time if they have managed to keep their job this long.

<u>Damage and Irrecoverable Phase</u>:

This is the third phase of caregiving. The span of this phase is between 37 months and 60 months.

This is the danger phase where the caregiver's health has deteriorated to a point where the caregiver is on antidepressants and sometimes tranquilizers. The caregiver in this phase has trouble sleeping (usually due to the concomitant decline in health), lack of focus and fatigue.

At this phase, if the caregiver is older, family members begin to recognize symptoms that are similar to dementia. It is common to hear a family member report, "My dad takes care of my mom who was diagnosed with dementia last year, but lately it seems like he is losing it too."

The caregiver is also unable to make good judgment or to ask for help. At this phase some caregivers begin to fall or suffer injury due to fatigue and a lack of sleep. The typical caregiver in this period would be failing and sometimes ask for help but refuses the help because he or she is too fatigued to be organized enough to accept the help. He or she may have enough money to pay for care at least for respite, but can't make a good decision because of poor judgment.

At this point, the caregiver may risk his or her own health as well as the quality of life of the care recipient not because he or she does not care, but because he or she is too fatigued or worried about the house being seen the way it is by the people who come to offer help.

It is at this point that institutional placement becomes a solution, but at a time that such a decision causes guilt. It is at this stage that other family members or friends intercede and find alternate solutions for care. Sometimes it is the discovery of the unkempt house during a time of hospitalization of the care recipient (when the caregiver stays at the hospital with the care recipient) that alerts the family and friends to the living conditions of the caregiver and the care recipient.

Possible solutions at this point include hiring in-home help or hospitalization. Without intervention, the caregiver may become a candidate for long term care as well.

Top Seven Warning Signs and Symptoms of Caregiver Stress AKA Caregiver Syndrome

1. **Denial**—When a caregiver is in denial, he/she may say things like, "I know Dad is going to get better really soon." Usually, denial is about the disease and the effects that the disease has on the person who has been diagnosed. The caregiver should be aware of the signs and symptoms of neglect, because denial can often lead to neglect when the family member believes that the care recipient is getting better soon, or is truly not affected by the disease in the same way that others are.
2. **Depression**—Depression begins to break your spirit and affects your ability to cope. Some caregivers who are suffering from depression say things like, "I don't care anymore." Many caregivers with severe cases of clinical depression do not always recognize the symptoms. Some attribute the feelings of fatigue, loss of energy, difficulty sleeping, irritability, mood swings, or difficulty concentrating as a normal part of being the family caregiver. This is why they do not seek help. Depression is also a risk factor for chronic conditions like heart disease, diabetes and cancer.
3. **Insomnia and Sleep Deprivation**—Lack of sleep can affect a caregiver's ability to

concentrate, especially at work. This poses safety issues, especially for employed caregivers who operate machinery. A study at Ohio State University showed that family caregivers who had a high level of responsibility had 55% or more incidence of sleeplessness. In the last decade, newer research is showing that lack of sleep heightens the risk of many illnesses such as heart disease, obesity and diabetes. According to a study cited in the *Journal of the American Medical Association (JAMA)*, one third of stressed-out caregivers who had a chronic disease died either shortly before or soon after their care recipients.

4. **Anger**—Some caregivers feel angry, usually towards the care recipient or others who are around them. Anger is sometimes directed towards the disease or about the fact that there may not be a cure. At other times, the caregiver is angry because those around him/her do not fully understand the situation.

5. **Social Isolation**—The caregiver withdraws from friends and co-workers. Sometimes the caregiver is not able to have friends over because they're uncomfortable or embarrassed by their caregiving responsibilities. Some caregivers would say things like, "I don't really care about going out or getting together with

my neighbors or church friends anymore. All they want to do is tell me what I should be doing."

6. **Anxiety**—Sometimes, the family caregiver will become anxious every day, worried if he or she has the resources to handle the demands of caregiving. For some caregivers, the thought that their loved ones disease may someday get worse causes them a lot of anxiety. Unfortunately, when the caregiver is anxious, the care recipient becomes anxious too. Anxiety also leads to lack of concentration, making it difficult for the caregiver to perform familiar and necessary tasks. During these times, caregivers will say things like, "I am too tired for anything" or "I am so busy that I forgot all about Dad's appointments."

7. **Health Problems**—Many family caregivers suffer from mental, emotional and physical health challenges. Heart disease, diabetes and cancer are the major health challenges facing family caregivers today. Usually by the second phase of caregiving (the exhaustion phase), the caregiver is already suffering from health challenges caused by prolonged stress or lack of self-care.

CHAPTER 4
DYING EARLY

*   *   *

24/7 Lifeline Tip #4

Respite is designed to ease the burden on family caregivers who must provide care for a person in need of extensive physical, mental, psychological, cognitive or emotional assistance and support. Most family caregivers get respite care only when there is a crisis. Waiting until a crisis happens before setting up respite care can cause you more stress because of the rush needed to get a plan in place.

*   *   *

THE ELDER CLIFF 1.0

A True Story: Caregiver Dies Shortly After Her Dear Mother

You have heard it said time and again, and you may have said it yourself: "I can't wait to take a vacation," or "Oh, I need a vacation bad!"

Upstairs in her bedroom, this lady was saying the very same thing as she pulled open her desk drawer that was loaded full of brochures that she had collected over the years. Brochures of every kind, from day trips to the casino across the state line, to 14-day cruises to Mexico and even trips to Europe. You name it, she had some literature for it.

A little out of breath, she tramped downstairs with a smile of hope as she poured everything from that drawer onto the coffee table. Over the years, she had picked up about 20 pounds—which her doctor had a lot to say about—so she was also contemplating shredding a few pounds before this vacation.

Carefully arranging the brochures according to the most colorful and the least expensive, she called her childhood friend and caregiving partner over for a discussion on the potential vacation spots. Together, they decided that they would make a dinner out of this vacation-finding event. So off to the steak house they went.

Sitting in the restaurant, showing their brochures of different vacation spots and collecting opinions from each waiter and all the people they dared to asked, they decided on a lavish $10,000 cruise to the Bahamas. Couldn't be any more deserving—after all, mom had just died after a long caregiving situation of some four years.

Mom left behind over half a million dollars, so $10,000 wasn't much. This was the only daughter. She had a brother who lived out of state, and he only visited once or twice a year to supervise and criticize.

Thanks to the strong daughter who had worked hard to care for mom by herself, as much as she could, while trying to hold down a full time job so she could hold on to the money in case mom got worse and needed the nursing home—or so she thought.

So picture this: mom passes away, and daughter's retirement rolls in that same month. What a perfect time for a caregiver to take a vacation and finally catch her breath. This daughter had worked hard and persevered through thick and thin, even as mom's health began to fail even more.

She deserved this vacation because between what she inherited from mom, her pension, and a huge check for all the vacation hours that she never took, she was sitting

The Elder Cliff 1.0

comfortably on a million dollars-plus worth of assets. Well, by the end of the great steak dinner, a decision was made, and off to the lavish 14-day cruise they went.

The first week on the cruise was spectacular, with lots of rest, good food, relaxation, spa treatments like you have never seen before, cute guys and all that a real cruise can offer.

Life was great until day #9. This well-rested girl began to feel sick. "Well," said the cruise nurse, "what can I get for your flu-like symptoms?" Together, they worked on a motion sickness remedy which seemed to help just a bit. She wanted to manage until she made it back home. Finally home, she thought she would be okay if she just rested for a few days. "I didn't realize how tired I was until I started to rest," she said.

Days passed but the fatigue and her discomfort would not go away. "Okay," she decided, "it's time to check in with the doctor and, oh my gosh, he is going to scream because my blood pressure is high, I haven't been there for a long time, and I have gained weight instead of losing it as we talked about on my last visit . . . and I don't even remember when that was."

With courage and no other way out, she went to the doctor's office. "I beg your pardon?" asked the doctor. "You have been sick for how long?"

"For about two weeks now," and she recounted the experiences of the cruise and the fact that she thought that she was just tired.

"Okay," the doctor nodded, "and how is your mother by the way?"

"Well, doctor," she replied, "you see, she died about six weeks ago and I finally decided to get away and take a break. I also retired right after her funeral, and now I want to just kick back and enjoy all the things that I have worked so hard for all these years. I sacrificed a lot," she explained to the doctor, "and did a lot to give her good care. I watched the money closely so it would last. I had help from a friend or two. Every now and then, she went to day care when I had work deadlines that I needed to meet."

She continued, "You see, I work downtown and the drive back and forth each day just got old so, when I had the chance to retire, I took it. But mom couldn't wait to enjoy it with me."

"I see," said the doctor. "We better run some tests. It looks like you had a bad case of the flu and maybe some food poisoning too. Let's see you again in a week, and in the meantime keep hydrated and get more rest."

The Elder Cliff 1.0

"Yes, doctor, and thanks for taking me in today," she said as she dragged herself out to her car. The week went by and the doctor had bad news. The caregiver was very sick—as in advanced cancer that had spread. Three weeks later, she passed away.

Now, here comes the once-or-twice-a-year visiting, unsolicited supervising and criticizing brother from out of state. He inherits mom's and sister's estates, making him an instant millionaire.

The moral of this story is that you can lose yourself and your life to caregiving unless you take time to rest, strive for work-life balance, and take care of yourself first.

Find ways to remember this: if you wear your body out, where are you going to live? No, stress does not have to kill you. Let the moral of this story move you to rediscover your life, reclaim your health, and know that being a good caregiver means caring for yourself first, so that you may be able to provide care for a long time.

It is for this reason that when you fly, the airlines will tell you that if you are flying with a child, you should put on your mask first before putting on the mask of the child. If not, you might be out and so will the child. In caregiving, the roles can sometimes be reversed, so caring for your parent can feel like caring for your child.

How Caregiver Stress Can Destroy You

You may have heard this before—that the caregiver dies either before or shortly after the care recipient. Every time I say this, I often well up in tears and so do the people who attend my caregiving seminars. If you are a family caregiver, *you are at a greater health risk than your loved one*. This is because by dedicating yourself and your resources to the needs of the other person you tend to neglect your own needs.

Science has proven what caregivers have talked about anecdotally for decades: that providing care to someone you care about and love takes a huge toll physically, emotionally, socially, and these days, financially. Many caregivers acknowledge that they are stressed, but they do not recognize the link between caregiving stress and what they are experiencing.

Over the past decade, a lot of research has shown that there is a significant link between caregivers' stress and poor health. Caregivers reported stress and stress-related chronic diseases and disorders at nearly twice the rate of non-caregivers.

Here are a few frightening statistics:

- According to the National Academy of Sciences, the stress of family caregiving for persons with

dementia has shown to impact a person's immune system for up to three years after their caregiving ends, thus increasing their chances of developing a chronic illness themselves.
- According to the National Alliance for Caregiving and a study by MetLife Insurance, approximately 32% of family caregivers report not going to the doctor as often as they should, and 55% say they skip doctor appointments for themselves.
- Sixty-three percent of caregivers report having poorer eating habits than non-caregivers, and 58% indicate worse exercise habits than they did before assuming their caregiving responsibilities.
- According to the MetLife study of family caregivers and employer health costs, 25% of employed female caregivers over 50 years old report symptoms of depression, compared to 8% of their non-caregiving peers.
- According to an assessment of family caregivers in 2006, up to 70% of family caregivers have clinically significant symptoms of depression, with approximately a quarter to half of these caregivers meeting the diagnostic criteria for major depression.
- In 2005, the Center on Aging Society reported that 1 in 10 of family caregivers reported that

caregiving had caused their physical health to deteriorate, while in 2012, 5 in 10 caregivers report the same.
- According to a National Academy of Science study in 2005, family caregivers experiencing extreme stress have been shown to age prematurely. This level of stress can reduce a caregiver's life span by as much as 10 years.
- In 2006, a study cited in the *New England Journal of Medicine* reported that a wife's hospitalization increased her husband's chances of dying within a month by 35%. A husband's hospitalization on the other hand raised his wife's mortality risk by 44%.

So why would your health go down when all you are trying to do is help?

Here is what the doctors are saying, and I believe them, too—because I preach it every day. Don't ignore this message! When you are stressed out, your body undergoes many physiological changes, most of which you can't feel and see. Since you don't generally get a warning from your body to slow down, you will just have to trust me and the doctors on this. Remember that your body is an amazing machine and it responds like this:

There is something called IL-6 protein. It is one of the proteins in the cytokine family. When you experience stress, the level of IL-6 rises. Based on a study of elderly caregivers, this level rises four times higher for those involved in caregiving. Part of the reason is that, as an individual ages, the normal levels of IL-6 in the body rises. Elevated levels of IL-6 in the body hinder how the immune system functions. Since caregivers' IL-6 levels increase four times higher than non-caregivers, caregivers are prone to a higher incidence of infections and illnesses, putting them at a greater risk for everything from colds to flu, heart diseases and cancer.

As a family caregiver, chances are that your health is suffering from the stress you face in your role as a caregiver. **So what is a caregiver to do when there is no one else to help?**

You have to find a way to take a break and to care for yourself so that you can continue to be a caregiver longer, and so that the person you are caring for will also continue to thrive. See **Chapter 6** for the different types of respite care and **Chapter 7** for where to get money to pay for respite care.

CHAPTER 5

MEASURING YOUR CAREGIVER STRESS

* * *

24/7 Lifeline Tip #5

Many older adults are lonely and isolated. An adult day care facility may help them find new friends and develop new experiences, which in turn helps them stay connected to the life around them. Most older adults become significantly improved with regular medical care, regular meals and a mentally stimulating environment. Most older adults who have trouble sleeping at night regain an improved nighttime sleep pattern once they attend an adult day care regularly. The physical activities and increased mobility cause them to be tired at the end of the day, and they sleep better. Improved quality of sleep improves the immune system and the ability to function better the next day. Caregivers who utilize adult day care services report more positive caregiving experiences.

* * *

The Caregiver Syndrometer

The **caregiver syndrometer** is a tool that I developed in 2009 based on my experience helping caregivers prevent collapse, breakdown or hospitalization. What I have learned is that most caregivers only speak up when they are in a crisis and call only when they are at their breaking point.

It is my hope that the caregiver syndrometer will be used by many caregivers and that it will help to reduce the number of care crashes—when the caregiver falls apart and the care recipient needs to be placed in a facility or hospital—that we see in the caregiving world.

The caregiver syndrometer measures how the stress caused by caregiving affects the life of the caregiver on five different dimensions:

1. physical wellbeing
2. emotional wellbeing
3. social wellbeing
4. financial strain
5. work/life balance

The total number of possible points for the meter is 100. The lower your total number of points or score, the better. A lower score indicates that you are a balanced caregiver and the likelihood of a care crash (when things fall apart) and poor health caused by caregiver stress is lower.

On the other hand, a higher score indicates that your life has been absorbed by caregiving and that your caregiver stress is higher indicating increased likelihood of dying either before or shortly after your care recipient.

The Caregiver Syndrometer	
100	Extreme Danger Zone
95	
90	
85	
80	
75	
70	
65	
60	
55	
50	Danger Zone
45	
40	
35	Caution Zone
30	
25	Realistic Balance in Caregiving
0	

The Caregiver Syndrometer

What Is the Level of Your Caregiver Stress?

In the caregiver syndrometer scoring checklist (below), some of the statements are worded to describe almost extreme situations, and some may not completely apply to you. Consider thinking deeply about **why even half of the statement applies to you** and consider taking steps to reduce the stress that you are going through.

- Place a check mark next to each item if the statement describes how you feel frequently. Each check mark is 4 points.
- Next, tally all the check marks.
- If the total number of points **exceeds 50**, then your health is at risk and your caregiving situation is at risk for a crash. **A score greater than 50 points is an indication that you should use respite services right away.**
- Consider contacting your doctor for a check-up, and then consulting a care manager for help with setting up a respite program for you and your care recipient.

THE ELDER CLIFF 1.0

The Caregiver Syndrometer Scoring Checklist

Physical Wellbeing:

___ He/she needs me to perform three or more activities of daily living.
___ I am physically tired.
___ I am not getting enough sleep.
___ I have to watch him/her constantly.
___ He/she is dependent on me for almost everything.

Emotional Wellbeing:

___ He/she is dependent on me.
___ I don't get along with others as well as I used to.
___ I resent my family members or friends for not helping.
___ I don't feel appreciated by my family.
___ I wish I could escape this situation.
___ I feel agitated or angry about my interactions with him/her.

Financial Strain:

___ I have had to change jobs so that I can provide care.
___ I have had to spend my own funds to pay for care related expenses.

___I have spent some of my money to pay for supplies.
___I have quit my job to provide care.
___I cannot save because I need to contribute to care expenses.

Work/Life Balance

___I feel uncomfortable when I have friends or co-workers over.
___I work a different schedule now so I can be at home for caregiving.
___I feel like I am missing out on life.
___This is not where I thought I would be at this time.

Social Wellbeing

___I don't enjoy going out any more.
___I feel like I am missing out on life.
___I have problems with my marriage or significant relationships.
___I feel isolated because he/she makes others uncomfortable.
___I am embarrassed over his/her behavior.

CHAPTER 6

WHAT IS RESPITE CARE?

* * *

24/7 Lifeline Tip #6

You may be eligible to receive a tax credit of up to 30% of the cost of adult day care, care management, care coordination and in-home care if you hire someone to take care of your loved one while you work. You will have to make the Social Security contributions on the person's behalf to qualify for this credit. Check with your accountant for the required documentation and tax details.

* * *

Respite simply means taking a break.

Respite care is temporary, short-term, coordinated, and supervised care provided to a care recipient with physical, mental or emotional impairments. Usually, respite care benefits both the caregiver and the care recipient. For the purpose of this book, respite care is the break from caregiving that the caregiver should be receiving.

There are a several types of respite care available so every caregiver should be able to use this help. Respite care is not the same in every state and county and varies, in part, on the availability of state or county funded services.

Respite can vary in time from part of a day to several weeks. Respite encompasses a wide variety of services including traditional home-based care, adult day care, skilled nursing home health care and short term institutional care.

The Three Most Common Types of Respite Care Services

The three most common types of respite stays are in-home care, adult day care, and short term institutional/assisted living care.

1. In-home Respite Care:

This is the most commonly used form of respite. Generally speaking, in-home respite care can be formal or informal.

Informal respite care is care provided by family members, friends, neighbors, or church volunteers who offer to stay with your elderly loved one while you go to the store or run other errands. Sometimes local church groups or councils on aging run "Friendly Visitor Programs" in which volunteers may be able to provide basic respite care, just like family members do. Many communities have formed either Interfaith Caregiver or Faith in Action programs where volunteers from faith-based communities are matched with caregivers to provide them with some relief. I encourage caregivers to seek these avenues, because not only do they provide good services, but most of them bring added value such as faith-based support to the care recipient.

Formal in-home care can be provided by companions, homemakers, personal care service aides, and skilled professionals like nurses.

2. Adult Day Care:

These are daytime recreational programs, some of which provide medically-oriented companionship and supervision. Adult day care programs offer relief to family members or caregivers, allowing them the freedom to go to work, handle personal business or just relax while knowing their relative is well cared for and safe. The advantages of Adult Day Care include peer group support, mental stimulation, personal care assistance and social interaction for the care receiver, while the caregiver obtains a "break" from caregiving responsibilities at less cost than in-home services.

3. Institutional/Assisted Living Short Term Stay:

This type of respite involves a short term stay for the care recipient at a long term care facility or at an assisted living facility. This usually begins with a level of care assessment. The purpose of the level of care assessment is to determine what type of care is needed to keep your loved one safe, comfortable, and thriving while you take a break. Assisted living services include housekeeping, laundry, meals, wellness checks, dressing, personal care, grooming, medication management, and symptom management.

Assisted living facilities are supervised and professionally equipped to handle emergencies, which alleviates family anxiety about care during planned respite stays for either a short weekend or an extended vacation.

Some family caregivers can also use this type of respite on a trial basis before permanent placement.

How to Find "Quality" Respite Care

When evaluating a respite care program or a respite facility, I encourage you to check to see if it is licensed by the state (where required), and if the caregivers have the qualifications necessary for professional caregiving. I have listed 12 questions that you can ask to assess credentials and qualifications.

1. Are families limited to a certain number of hours for services needed?
2. Can the provider take care of more than one person at a time?
3. Can family members meet and interview the people who will be providing the respite care?
4. Does the program provide transportation for the care recipient?
5. Does the program keep an active file on the care recipient's medical condition and other needs? Is there a written care plan?
6. How are the caregivers screened?
7. How are the caregivers trained? Do they receive extra training, where appropriate, to meet the specific family needs of the care recipient and the family?

8. How are the caregivers supervised and evaluated?
9. How much does the respite care cost? What is included in the fee?
10. How far ahead of time do family members need to call to arrange services?
11. How does the provider or facility handle emergencies? What instructions do they receive to prepare them for unexpected situations like an emergency evacuation?
12. How is the program evaluated? Are family members contacted for their feedback? If so, ask if you can review their comments!

Questions to Ask and What to Look for When Hiring a Private In-Home Caregiver

For purposes of this section, a private in-home caregiver is someone who works for him or herself and is not working through a bonded and insured home health agency. When interviewing an in-home respite care aide, you may want to ask the following questions:

- Are you insured?
- Do you have any references? What are they?
- Do you have any special skills that would help you with this job?

- Have you ever worked with someone in the same medical condition as my loved one?
- How would you handle the following situation? (Cite examples of challenges you have encountered as a family caregiver.)
- What is your background and training?
- What are your past experiences in providing respite care?
- When are you available? Do you have a back-up/assistant if you are unable to come when expected?
- Why are you interested in this job?
- Why did you leave your last job?

CHAPTER 7

TEN PLACES TO GET MONEY AND RESOURCES FOR RESPITE CARE

* * *

24/7 Lifeline Tip #7

Hospice care is not only for those who are experiencing imminent death. Hospice care is also for people with a life limiting disorder. Hospice care is a plan for living when you have a life limiting disorder. Hospice services can also be beneficial to the family members of the care recipient through grief support services. Grief counseling and bereavement counseling is available for up to one year after the death of the care recipient.

* * *

The Elder Cliff 1.0

This is a tricky subject especially when you have spent months or years asking your parents or loved one about their financial situation, and every time you ask, you are told to "mind your own business," "don't worry about us," or "we didn't want to be a burden to anybody" and the like. It can be even more difficult when you do not have all the correct documents, such as general or durable power of attorney that you will need to access your loved one's financial records or bank account. Whatever your situation, there are 10 places to find money to pay for respite care.

1. Respite Reimbursement Grants

These grants are federal dollars that come through the National Family Caregiver Support Program. You do not have to repay them nor do you have to pay taxes on them. To get a respite reimbursement grant, call your local Area Agency on Aging (this agency is different from the Council on Aging) and ask for the Family Caregiver Support Program. Each agency administers the program differently, but the bottom line is that you can have free respite care if you meet the requirements. Ninety percent (90%) of family caregivers qualify for these grants. It is usually not based on income, but income can influence the amount of respite reimbursement that you receive.

With some programs, the caregiver gets reimbursed for respite care that the caregiver pays for, while in other programs, the Family Caregiver Support Program pays the respite provider directly through pre-existing contracts. Some of these grants range in value from $500.00 up to $24,000.00. I have seen this program reimburse a family for two and a half months of around-the-clock respite care.

You can visit the National Family Caregiver Support Program at http://www.aoa.gov/AoARoot/AoA_Programs/HCLTC/Caregiver/index.aspx.

2. The Alzheimer's Association Substitute Family Caregiver Program

The Alzheimer's Association has a program called the Substitute Caregiver Program. Some chapters administer this program like the National Family Caregiver Support Program, where you, the caregiver, are reimbursed for respite care. In most cases, the care recipient has to have a diagnosis of memory loss to qualify for this program. To learn more, visit www.AlzheimersAssociation.org.

3. The Local Council on Aging

This service is different from the local Area Agency on Aging. Most councils on aging have the Title III federal funds to use for respite services for family members. Respite care through most councils on aging respite services range from homemaker services, companionship, personal care and transportation. Sometimes their services are free, although they are limited in the amount of care they provide.

4. Meals on Wheels

Meals on Wheels as respite care? I include it here because Meals on Wheels can save the family caregiver from having to cook all the required meals. For those family caregivers who don't have any assistance, having someone provide a hot lunch and a bedtime snack can provide an hour or two of rest. Sometimes, an hour or two of rest is what the family caregiver needs to restore and refresh him or herself.

5. The Basement, Attic and Garage Sale

It may sound like a stretch—but stick with me. Put the book down and go open the garage, the basement or even the attic. There are items in there that can be sold and the money used for respite care. You are going to need to clean out the house and hold a garage sale later on anyway, so why not do it now and use the money toward care?

6. Cut Back on the Pharmacy Bill

No, I am not talking about not refilling some of the prescriptions. I am talking about asking the doctors to prescribe generics when possible, so you can save on the pharmacy expenses. You can then take the money you have saved and put it toward respite care.

Here is another example: 80 mg tablets of the water pill called Lasix are less expensive than the 40 mg tablets. If the doctor orders 80 mg prescribed at ½ a tablet, you still have the correct dose but at a lesser price. What about asking the doctor to look at all the medications, and cut back on whatever can be cut back? Or, see if you can get a combination medication such as one med for both cholesterol and hypertension. In fact, you might notice that your loved one does better on fewer medications.

7. Cut Back on the Personal Care Bill

Family caregivers report that personal care items take up to 25% of the care budget. Take for example the cost of disposable undergarments. There is a brand called Tranquility All-Through-The-Night. This undergarment can hold up to one gallon of fluid without leaking. Better yet, these Tranquility undergarments are odor free and keep the skin dry even for the person who is severely incontinent. There are polymers inside of this garment which are antimicrobial and form a gel when urine touches the undergarment, which is why those who use them do not experience urine odor or urinary infections like those who use other brands. If you are spending $50 to $75 a month on disposable undergarments, you can save about 30% of that cost by switching to the Tranquility brand. That alone can provide 20-30 respite care days per year for a family. Where can you find these undergarments? Try the Home Health Care Supply Outlet at www.homecaresupplyoutlet.com or call **440-266-1770** for samples.

8. The Veteran's Administration

The Veteran's Administration is one of the best places to get free respite care. Of course, the care recipient has to be a veteran to enjoy this benefit. The best way to access this benefit is to go to the main Veteran's Administration hospital closest to your home and register for services. Sometimes it takes several weeks to get an appointment at a local VA hospital. If you are stressed and can't wait, then go into the emergency room and through the emergency services, and you will be able to obtain a social worker appointment.

Your loved one will also need to be registered for general medicine with the Veteran's Administration.

They do not need to completely change doctors but must have a Veteran's Administration medical file to access some of their services. The VA will pay for approximately 14 hours of respite care per week at no charge to most vets. These services are provided by agencies that have specific relationships with the VA. It takes approximately 2-6 weeks to set up respite care through a VA service provider. The VA also pays for up to 30 days per year of respite care in a facility such as an Assisted Living Facility or a nursing home.

9. Barter Your Time

To work for respite care sounds a little crazy. Here I am telling you how you need a break and then I am also saying that you should work to get a break? Not everybody needs to work outside of the home to feel refreshed. But for some people, having a job or volunteering can provide a change of environment, a break, or relaxation away from the usual day-in, day-out caregiving situation. Sometimes, caregivers can volunteer for an organization (adult day care, a church) in exchange for respite care.

10. Hospice Care

This can be a really good option for someone whose loved one has a life limiting disorder. This is not the kind of hospice care when death is imminent. This can be a plan for living when your loved one has any of the following indicators:

- Multiple falls
- Increased assistance with activities of daily living
- Skin integrity or skin break down, also commonly known as bed sores
- Multiple fractures
- Weight loss
- Changes in mental status
- Multiple visits to the emergency room
- Multiple medications
- Increasing shortness of breath

Once any of the above listed indicators reach a certain level of severity or frequency, these symptoms may indicate that palliative hospice care should be considered.

CHAPTER 8

THE FIVE COMPONENTS OF A GOOD RESPITE PLAN

* * *

24/7 Lifeline Tip #8

Your emotional relationship with your family member will change. Sometimes, older adults experience emotional difficulties or behave strangely partly because of the medications that they are taking. Your care recipient's ability to change is extremely limited and may diminish as their disease progresses. Check with the doctors to discover possible organic causes of depression and/or behavioral changes. You (not your love one) will have to change. This means that you will have to learn to accept their behavior and learn how to alter your expectations and adjust your reactions.

* * *

One of the difficulties of being the caregiver is the element of role reversal. This becomes a major issue when respite care is involved because when you are an adult child or a spouse playing the role of the caregiver, it may sometimes feel like your loved one is a child again.

As you build a respite plan, focus on only two things:

1. Focus on the fact that, for you to continue to be an available caregiver, you have to take a break. View respite care as an investment into your loved one's long term care.
2. Focus on the fact that your loved one will benefit from the interaction with the respite provider. Plus, in the event of an emergency, you can use the respite care as your backup plan.

A solid respite plan should have the following five components:

#1: Flexibility

Your respite service provider should have some degree of flexibility in service, in case your loved one has "good days" and "bad days." The provider should be able to provide respite in four-hour blocks or more. This will make it possible for your loved one to receive care if or when he or she can only tolerate a short time of care/activity.

#2. Availability of Emergency Medical Services

The respite provider should have a system of obtaining and managing emergency medical services so that your loved one will have access to adequate medical care in an emergency.

#3. Medically Superior and Medically Oriented Care

It is amazing how the human body can change. All of a sudden, your loved one can become incontinent. Your respite provider should be able to handle incontinence and personal care so that when that time comes, your loved one does not need to change providers. By the way, you will need to leave a complete change of clothing in case your loved one has a personal care accident and needs clean clothing.

#4. Access to a Caregiving Referral Network

Nothing about elder care is easy and no two situations are the same. Every day presents its own challenges, and the need for other services comes up quite frequently. A good respite plan should include the resourcefulness and ability to access all the other needed eldercare services. A good one-stop shop for "everything eldercare" is The National Care Planning

Council. You can reach them by visiting their website at www.longtermcarelink.net.

#5. Cost Effective

Of course, I saved the best for last. Since the downturn of the economy, the cost of health care has been on the rise all over the country.

- The national average daily rate for private, custodial care in a long term facility like a nursing home rose over 4% in the past two years, from $229 per day in 2010 to $239 per day in 2012.
- In assisted living, costs rose almost 6% from $3293 per month in 2010 to $3477 per month in 2012.
- Adult day care costs rose also, but generally it is still the most cost effective objective for respite care. The national average rate for 8-12 hours of adult day care services is $61.00 per day.
- In-home care, on the other hand, is $19.00 per hour for non-medical care.

You will want the most cost effective care for your situation so that you can take as much respite time as possible.

Where Can I Learn More About Respite Services?

The following organizations provide useful information to caregivers on a variety of topics including respite:

ARCH National Respite Network and Resource Center

This organization works to ensure all family caregivers have access to quality respite. The mission of the ARCH National Respite Network is to assist and promote the development of quality respite and crisis care programs; to help families locate respite and crisis care services in their communities; it serves as a strong voice for respite in all forums.

ARCH Website: http://www.archrespite.org/

Phone: 703-256-2084

ARCH National Respite Locator Service: http://www.respitelocator.org/

The Alzheimer's Association

The Alzheimer's Association provides education and support for people diagnosed with the condition, their families, and caregivers. To find a local chapter closest to you or to order a copy of the association's respite care guide, visit their website at http://www.alz.org or call 800-272-3900.

The Family Caregiver Alliance

The Family Caregiver Alliance runs a resource center and publishes fact sheets and a newsletter with tips for family caregivers. The organization can be reached by calling 1-415-434-3388 or visiting its website at: http://www.caregiver.org

The National Alliance for Caregiving

The National Alliance for Caregiving is a joint venture of several private and governmental agencies. The alliance website provides useful information and links for caregivers. You can contact this resource by visiting its website at: http://www.caregiving.org

National Adult Day Services Association

Information concerning adult day services can be obtained from the National Adult Day Services Association at (703) 610-9005 or by visiting their website at: http://www.nadsa.org

To find out more about hospice programs where you live, you can contact your local aging information and assistance provider or Area Agency on Aging (AAA). **The Eldercare Locator**, a public service of the Administration on Aging (at 1-800-677-1116 or http://www.eldercare.gov) can help connect you to these agencies.

CHAPTER 9

CARING FOR YOURSELF SO YOU DON'T DIE EARLY

* * *

24/7 Lifeline Tip #9

Life is Now, Today is for Gratitude. Look for the "present" in today. No matter how challenging today may be, find something—even if it is just a little thing to be grateful for—because tomorrow may never come, and if does, it could be worse. There is a present for you today; look for it, look closer, look with hope, look with gratitude.

* * *

The Elder Cliff 1.0

Each person is different and each family is different. What works for one person may not work for another person. What is relaxing to one person may not be relaxing to another person. Here is an example: I once asked a client of mine what her idea of respite was, and here is what she wrote:

> "The way you describe respite sounds refreshing and wonderful. My pocket book determines most of what I do, which is a shame. For me, respite would be to go to Seattle where my two grown children live. My granddaughter is a senior this year at North Bend Academy and I have never seen her play high school basketball. Now for what I could afford, I love to read and I love to take my book to a coffee shop and grab a scone and to just sit there and read. It is quite relaxing and just makes me feel better. Just the little things, and as you always say, just look for the moments. Sitting with my book and a cup of coffee helps me relax, it makes me feel good and collect the moments."—Annie B.

Me, I would have done the exact opposite. My idea of a day of respite would have been to go for a walk, sit under a tree, watch nature, and get some ice cream and dry roasted peanuts (no salt by the way) and wash it down with a tall bottle of Mountain Dew. I am thankful for small blessings and small peaceful moments.

For somebody else, it is a small peace island. A peace island is simply a place in which you can feel at peace. It can just be a matter of feeling peace and having peace only in your mind and your body. You could even have an actual place that you make as a peace island. You could select a spot where you can move around easily, allowing you to utilize all of your senses. It could be a small corner of your den, a little table in your back yard, a corner of your patio or even an end table right in the middle of your living room. The goal of a peace island is to **create a place that allows you to be at ease**—to get into a peaceful mode naturally and or physically. Your island should be a place where you can smell, feel, hear, see and touch the things that can bring you into a state of relaxation and complete peacefulness.

If you choose to make a peace island, here are a few things that you can use:

(1) Something that you can smell (a relaxing candle)
(2) Something you can see (maybe a small table fountain)
(3) Something you can hear (like soft music)
(4) Something you can touch (some art work or clay, or a stress ball)
(5) Something that you can feel (maybe dipping your hands in paraffin wax or sitting on a chair with a back massager)

Whatever will let you relax and feel at peace would make for a good peace island.

The Top 10 Ways to Care for Yourself

Another good way to think about this is **10 ways to invest in the quality of life of your care recipient**. Preferably, do more than one action a day, but at least do one every other day. Make it a priority to take care of yourself, and you will become a better caregiver in the process.

#1. Ask for help.

Begin with the universe, your creator God, or whomever represents your higher power. If you have other family members, suggest a plan. Divide up responsibilities and caregiving tasks. If you have long distance family members, find out how they can contribute toward respite care. If you do not have family, seek out and use community resources both for you and your care recipient.

#2. Accept help.

Sometimes the strongest thing you can do is to ask for help. Help is a tool, not a weakness. Help is an essential tool needed for you to become a more effective and more resourceful caregiver. Make it a daily goal to accept some kind of help. Consider that help as an investment into your caregiver's life.

#3. Exercise.

It does not have to be a whole hour of aerobics with all the coordinated gear and the perfect cross training shoes. That can be complicated or impossible when you don't have even 20 minutes to yourself. Just five minutes of exercise while sitting in your living room watching television could do much good for your body. Even five minutes of stretching can do wonders for back health and stress management.

#4. Eat well.

A balanced meal can sound like a luxury sometimes, but a good diet is essential for the management of stress and fatigue. Avoid highly concentrated sweets or sugar foods. Sometimes after a long, hard day, a sugary snack may feel like a reward. If that is the case, then make it a small portion, enjoy it, savor it and then eat some good protein like nuts to keep the body on an even keel all day.

#5. Take a break every day—Respite.

Imagine that you had to hold a half gallon of milk above your head for several days straight. If you were given an opportunity to put it down every 15 minutes, you could possibly do this for weeks and years without end, because every 15 minutes, you get to rest. That is exactly how respite care serves you. If you take a break every day you will be a balanced and successful caregiver for a long time. It does not have to be a long, planned out, complicated respite service. Just stop and rest and take a break so that you can be recharged.

#6. Music.

Listen to music and spend time in your peace island. Research has shown that music has a way of reaching the subconscious and bringing back memories. Find music that relaxes you or speaks to your situation. Something to help you unwind, recharge, and inspire.

#7. Talk to someone every day.

You can maintain your role as a caregiver longer if you are able to share your thoughts, fears, feeling and frustration with others. With today's online community, there are many blogs and online support groups that help caregivers connect to share their experiences.

Medicare did an Alzheimer's project for family caregivers where it was discovered that caregiver support groups and caregivers' connections were one of the top ways that caregivers survive and cope in their caregiving roles.

#8. Know your limits.

Be realistic with yourself about what you can do, what feels acceptable and what is comfortable for you. Guilt has a way of playing against a caregiver's ability to maintain boundaries. Keep in mind that other caregivers often have different roles and responsibilities than you, so doing what others do is not a healthy approach. Consider your work/life balance. Check your caregiver syndrometer. Use it as a gauge to measure your stress.

#9. Get adequate sleep.

When caring for someone with memory loss, you tend to sleep with one eye open and one ear open. Getting adequate sleep can be difficult at times. Eating a bowl of cereal with milk before sleep helps to promote a better quality of sleep. Foods higher in magnesium such as milk and peanut butter help to switch the body into sleep mode.

#10. Take it a day at a time.

Give yourself permission to cry. Caregiving has been nicknamed the "roller coaster from hell" because there are good days and bad days. Each event in life is natural—so when things are bad, and that day is going all wrong, embrace it all. Bad days do not make you a bad caregiver. Every day will come with its own challenges. If and when you are frustrated, give yourself permission to cry. When you cry, it does not mean that you are weak. It means that your heart is overflowing, and so are your eyes. Crying is therapeutic so allow yourself this relief. It is a very good way of relieving stress.

The Thriving Caregiver's Declaration

I want you to make the commitment to care for yourself so you will survive and thrive in caregiving. This declaration is for you and you only. No one has to see it, and no one needs to witness it with you. Use it as you may, and share it only when you are ready.

If you can't have long periods of respite time, then try five minutes each hour and by the end of the day, you will have succeeded in taking some time off to care for yourself.

THE THRIVING CAREGIVER'S DECLARATION

I am _____ caregiver, AKA an invisible hero of the family. On this _____ day of _____, 20___, I am writing to declare my SUPPORT to MYSELF for taking steps toward my self care.

I acknowledge the fact that in Caregiving, Love Is Not Enough, and accepting help and respite is an investment in myself, in the quality of life of my loved one, and in my role as a caregiver.

I intend to thrive as a caregiver by making a commitment to respite care and self care.

I will strive for 7 hours of respite care each day, even if I only collect them 5 minutes at a time.

A moment at a time, a day at a time, I intend to care for myself and to thrive.

Signed: _____

Witness_____

Witness_____

MAY YOU BE WELL AND THRIVE AS A CAREGIVER

… CHAPTER 10

THE ROLE OF CARE MANAGEMENT IN CAREGIVING

* * *

24/7 Lifeline Tip #10

Successful Caregiving is like a three-legged stool: the care recipient, the professionals and the Caregiving services available. All three legs must be present and stable for balanced Caregiving.

* * *

This chapter introduces you to care management and the role that a care manager can play in your caregiving situation. Usually, there is a fee for this service. In times of crisis, especially in long distance caregiving, a care manager can save you a lot of time, energy and stress.

When you do not know what else to do or how to get out from under your mountain of stress, reach out for a care manager. He or she will help sort through the complex situation and help get things under control very quickly.

The Top 10 Ways a Care Manager Can Help with Respite Care

1. Conduct a level of care assessment to identify caregiving problems and recommend caregiving solutions.
2. Provide crisis intervention in the home, at a hospital or at a care facility.
3. Screen, match and arrange for in-home help or other caregiving services, including assistance in hiring qualified caregivers at home.
4. Function as a liaison to families who are far away and even those who are close by for overseeing, coordinating and responding to family members in the event of a caregiving problem.

5. Facilitating the relocation of an older adult to and from a retirement community, assisted living facility or nursing home.
6. Provide advocacy and eldercare education to families and other care team members.
7. Provide eldercare counseling and support.
8. Review financial, legal and medical issues, and offer referrals to all appropriate medical and care specialists.
9. Provide financial, legal and medical review and assessments for the application of benefits, including Veterans Administration Aid and Attendance benefits, long term care insurance, and state medical waivers.
10. Help family members keep SANE and to find MEANING and JOY as they juggle responsibilities in all their caregiving roles.

The Three Best Places to Find Qualified Care Managers

1. National Care Planning Council

www.longtermcarelink.net

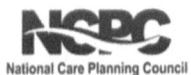

2. National Association of Professional Geriatric Care Managers

   www.caremanager.org

   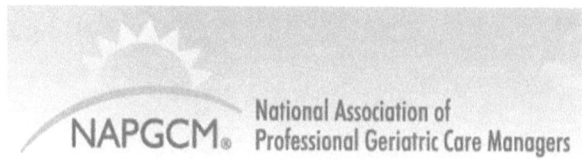

3. National Academy of Certified Care Managers

   www.NACCM.net

   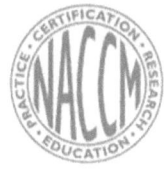

CHAPTER 11

"DONE FOR YOU" RESPITE CARE PLAN

* * *

24/7 Lifeline Tip #11

Make respite a part of your care plan. Plan for it and budget for it like you do an insurance premium, because respite is the premium you pay for balanced Caregiving.

* * *

The goal of a respite plan is to care for you so that you can continue to care. Respite is not just time to relax and pamper yourself. It is more than that. It is more than relaxing and "me time," as some of my clients would say. Respite is an investment into your health and your life, and that of the person that you are caring for. It is a necessity. Strive for at least seven hours a day or at minimum, seven hours a week.

There are three keys to a successful respite plan.

1. Be informed and keep informed.

The very first thing is to determine how much time, money, and resources you have that you can use towards respite care. You will have an idea about this when you have explored some or all of the 10 places to get money and resources for respite care (see Chapter 7).

Money is important, but you can take time for respite even if you do not have a lot of money to spend. Learn about the available community resources and services in your area. Visit health fairs and get on the mailing list for your community senior newsletter so that you will know what is happening and what you can take advantage of.

2. Share your caregiving responsibility.

Encourage as much independence in your care recipient as possible, and involve them in decisions about their care as long as they are able to participate. Involve your family and friends as much as possible. Don't wait for them to read your mind and offer help. Ask for help and think of "asking for help" as the strongest thing that you are doing. Be realistic when discussing this with your family members about what you can do and cannot do.

3. Manage your emotions.

Accept that frustration, anger, and sadness may come with caregiving—and you should try your best to accept these emotions without guilt. Grieving is quite normal. You may be grieving the loss of the active, well, and strong person in your memories as you care for a frail parent or relative. If you feel out of control, get some professional help. It comes with the territory and it is also an investment in caregiving. If you have to get professional help, tell the counselor that you are investing in your health and that of the person that you are caring for. You will be surprised by how much help you can get by saying it that way.

Respite Plan When You Have Less Than $100 per Month in Your Respite Budget

Strive for seven hours a day or seven hours a week of respite time for you.

$100 can go a little way if you plan it just right. Here is an idea. Try Meals on Wheels so that you can save yourself an hour a day from not preparing lunch or an afternoon snack. If you have to pay for it based on what Meals on Wheels may cost, you will have some money left over. Not cooking three meals out of the week can save you almost seven hours of time. The question is, what can you do if you had seven hours to yourself? You will have to be organized so that you can actually recognize the seven hours.

The other thing that you can do is make several meals ahead of time and put them in the freezer so that you do not spend too much time in the grocery store or the kitchen. Make your own homemade TV dinner and then sit in front of the TV and relax and have some "you time."

You will have to plan ahead so that you can get away and actually enjoy the seven hours. If you decide to do Meals on Wheels, you can get a neighbor to come over and check on your loved one and make sure that they actually did eat, so you can go out for a walk or go to the coffee house and sit and read a book by the fire place, if that is what you enjoy for "you time." If you enjoy a massage, go to a school of massage therapy and offer to be a guinea pig so the students can practice on you.

Your Respite Plan in Checklist Form

Select the option(s) that suits you best and find ways to work up to seven hours a day or seven hours a week. Perfection is not necessary. If you cannot get a whole hour by yourself, try for half an hour. It adds up and it counts.

- ___ Order Meals on Wheels at least three times a week.
- ___ Make five dinners ahead of time and freeze them.
- ___ Plan for a friend to come over and visit and serve as a companion.
- ___ Plan a getaway such as to a coffee house, a movie, a school of massage therapy, or get a pedicure.
- ___ Plan a walk with a good friend, or just walk and you might meet a stranger who might end up becoming a friend or another support system for you.

___ Attend a support group, chat on line or participate in a blog.
___ Take a nap an hour each day.
___ Journal, or just call up a friend.

Respite Plan When You Have $350 or More a Month in Your Respite Budget

The best use of $350.00 can be a combination of the following options.

Your Respite Plan in Checklist Form

___ Plan for adult day care for half a day, twice a week.
___ Take a nap one of the days that your loved one is gone to adult day care.
___ If adult day care is too much, try four hours of in-home respite at least once a week, and then you can get away.
___ Make some meals ahead of time and freeze them so you can enjoy a few hours in front of the TV or in a little quiet place (or in your peace island) a few times a week.
___ Attend a support group.
___ Go to the gym for half an hour twice a week.
___ Get a massage.
___ Get a pedicure or a manicure.

___ Write in your journal.
___ Go to a counselor.
___ Go to that doctor's appointment that your have cancelled a few times already.

Tips about Respite Options

If you have the choice of doing in-home respite or adult day care, choose adult day care. Why? It costs less so you get more care for your money, it is better for your loved one to be mentally stimulated by other people, and it will help your loved one physically if he or she is able to walk around inside an adult day center. The walking helps improve muscle tone, and the improved muscle tone will increase the mobility and functionality of your loved one. Here is a secret. If your loved one does not sleep well at night, the activities in an adult day center will help to tire him/her out and that will help reset the sleep pattern.

CHAPTER 12

THE SIX STEPS TO MAKING DECISIONS IN CAREGIVING: THE W.E.C.A.R.E. MODEL

* * *

24/7 Lifeline Tip #12

Nothing in eldercare is simple. No decision will be perfect. The key to making effective decisions is your willingness to analyze the risks versus the benefits of each situation.

* * *

The W.E.C.A.R.E. Model: The Wheel to Drive Your Caring Situation

W.E.C.A.R.E. is a decision making model that I have developed over the last 2 decades. It stands for:

Welcome professional services

Engage the care recipient

Create care options

Act on an option

Reassess the situation

Enhance independence

I call it W.E.C.A.R.E. because the most effective care plans are those that involve the caregiver, the care recipient, their wishes, their strengths and their need to feel alive and to enjoy more life out of days than days out of life. Many families have used this system in different degrees for different situations. It has one goal: To give the best care possible in the situation that you find yourself.

Imagine the caregiver at the center of a wheel. Around the CARE wheel should be:

1. Welcome professional services to give you an objective picture of the situation.
2. Engage the care recipient and discover their wishes.
3. Create realistic care options around the care recipient's wishes.
4. Act on an option.
5. Reassess the situation and the outcomes of the care option that you have acted upon.
6. Enhance independence to the extent possible.

The CARE Wheel

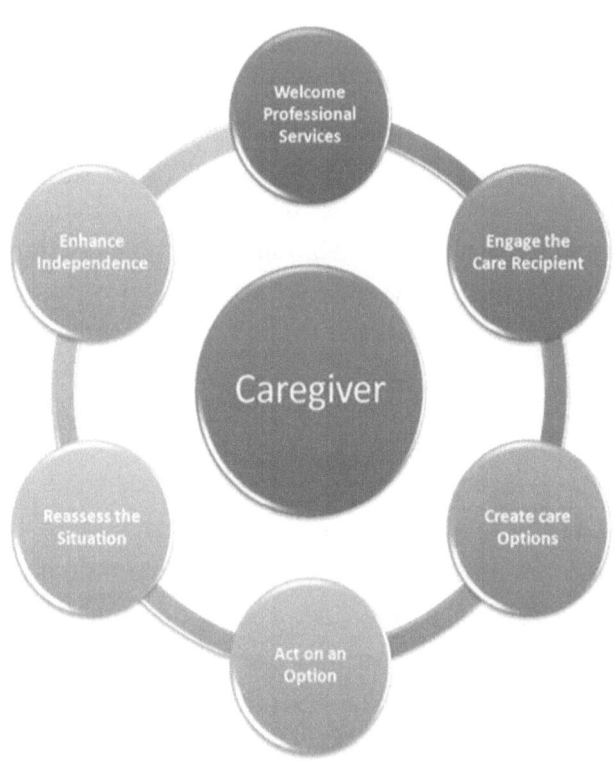

Three Tips for Making Successful Decisions in Caregiving

1. Allow your parents to take some risk.

It is natural to want to overprotect your parent especially when he or she is getting frail. However, that is usually the last thing an older person wants or needs. Too much protection can undermine your parent's self-esteem. The goal is to try for a balance in caring. Allow your parents to continue to carry out functions that they can still do even if with difficulty. If you take everything away, that may cause resistance, depression and dependence.

2. Safety should be first, not everything.

Safety is important but it is not the only thing. It is just as important to focus on the remaining abilities of your parents, as it is to focus on the limitations. You want to avoid forcing your values on your parents. What you think is best may not always be true. Very often, adult children are concerned with the parent's "quantity of life" but the parent is concerned with "quality of life."

3. Avoid promises. You may not be able to live up to them.

Try not to make promises like:

> *"I will never put you in a nursing home."*
> *"You can always live with us."*
> *"You can always stay in your home."*
> *"I will quit my job and take care of you if you need me to."*

What may seem like the best solution today may not be the same ten years from now when your own health or that of your parent has changed. Unfulfilled promises often result in guilt, anger, mistrust and disappointment.

Beware of the "Shoulds"

Also, watch out for the "shoulds" in caregiving. These usually come from guilt. If your parent's health deteriorates, you may find yourself with "shoulds" like these:

- A caring daughter should invite her parents to move in with her.
- A good son should not allow his mother to live alone.

- A responsible child should quit her job to care for her parents.

"Shoulds" may come from guilt within you, from other family members, from outside the family, from your parent's friends or from people who should not even matter like the mail carrier or the neighbor's house keeper. It's important not to let the guilt of "shoulds" guide your decisions.

Guilt can create very destructive outcomes: end a career, destroy a marriage, destroy mental health, destroy physical health or even sacrifice healthy relationships. Guilt can reduce objectivity, reduce your ability to decide on what is best for you, your parents and your family.

If a promise you are unable to keep is the source of "shoulds" guilt, anger and frustrations, look back at the conditions under which you made those promises and compare the situation of today. Most likely, the conditions are very different. Comparing *what is* with *what was* may help to give you clarity and an objective look at the current situation. That might make it easier for you to let go of a promise that is now completely unrealistic to keep. Forgive yourself and focus on the here and the now.

FINAL NOTE

May you live well, be present in your life today and may you thrive as you strive for moments of respite on a daily basis. I hope you will join me in the *Elder Care Cliff 2.0*. Meanwhile, claim your free report on *How To Get The Government To Pay Family Caregivers* at www.StellaNsong.com.

ABOUT THE AUTHOR

Stella Nsong, RN, CMC, CDP, LTCP

Care Manager Certified
Certified Dementia Practitioner
Long Term Care Planner

http://www.stellansong.com/

AUTHOR: Stella Nsong is a certified geriatric care manager and a certified dementia practitioner. She has been a nurse for more than twenty years and has worked in almost every branch of health care. Over fifteen years ago, she became a business owner and has owned, created, started, turned around, licensed, and managed private duty home care agencies, Medicare certified agencies, Medicaid certified agencies, medical adult day care centers, medical alert system companies, home medical supply companies, and assisted living facilities. A widely renowned public speaker and business success mentor, she has authored three books on eldercare and is a coauthor of the Gratitude Project for 2013. She is also the writer and editor of the Elder

Care Cliff Report. In 1990, she won the gold medal for practical nursing in the state of Georgia. In 2010, she was nominated Business Woman of the year in Chesterland, Ohio. In 2012, she was nominated for the Platinum Award in Care Management as well as The Professional of Note in Geriatric Medicine.

www.ingramcontent.com/pod-product-compliance
Lightning Source LLC
Chambersburg PA
CBHW022007170526
45157CB00003B/1181